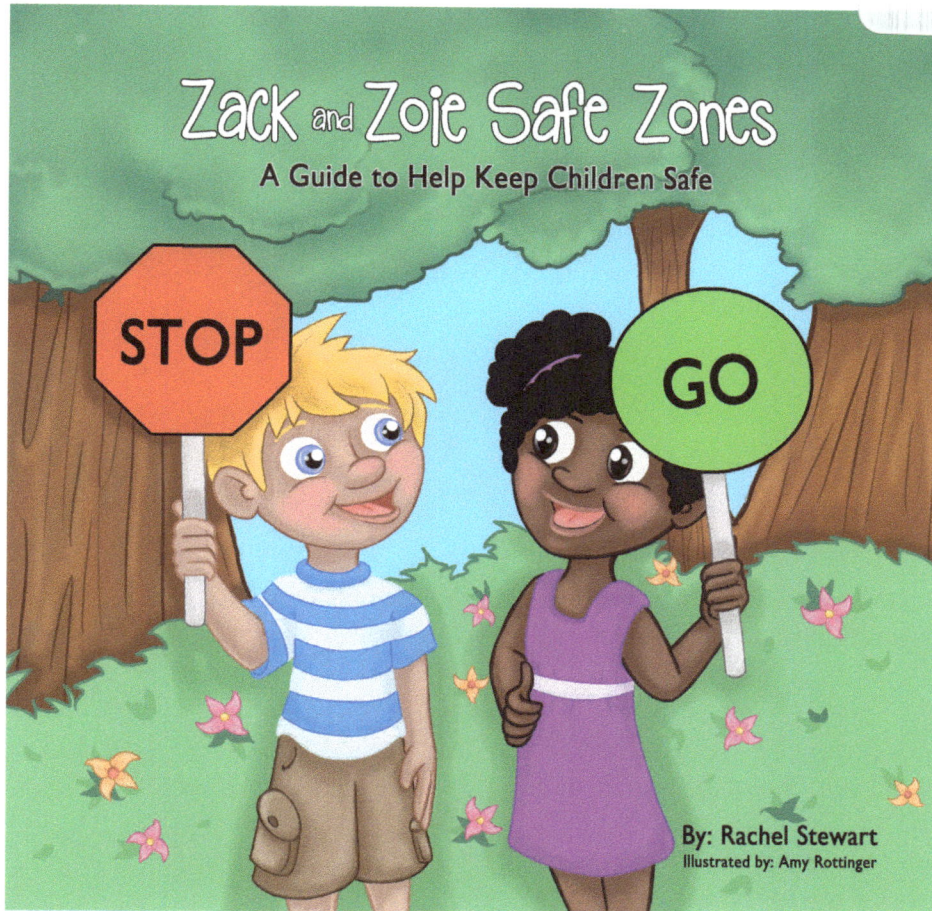

Zack and Zoie Safe Zones

A Guide to Help Keep Children Safe

By: Rachel Stewart

Illustrated by: Amy Rottinger

Halo ●●●●
Publishing International

Disclaimer:
Zack and Zoie Safe Zones: A Guide to Help Keep Children Safe is intended as an educational tool and does not guarantee the absence of abuse victimization.

ISBN 13: 978-1-61244-321-8
Library of Congress Control Number: 2014917659

Printed in the United States of America

Halo
Publishing International
www.halopublishing.com

Published by Halo Publishing International
1100 NW Loop 410
Suite 700 - 176
San Antonio, Texas 78213
Toll Free 1-877-705-9647
www.halopublishing.com
www.holapublishing.com
e-mail: contact@halopublishing.com

I would like to dedicate this book to all the children of the world who have the right and ability to keep safe. I want to thank God, my wonderful family, and friends for believing in the blessing of this book. I'm so grateful for my wonderful husband for his endless support. Many thanks to my sister for illustrating the original Zack and Zoie Safe Zones. Most of all, thank you to those who devote their lives to helping children.

Hello, my name is Zack. Hi, my name is Zoie. We are going to teach you something very important.

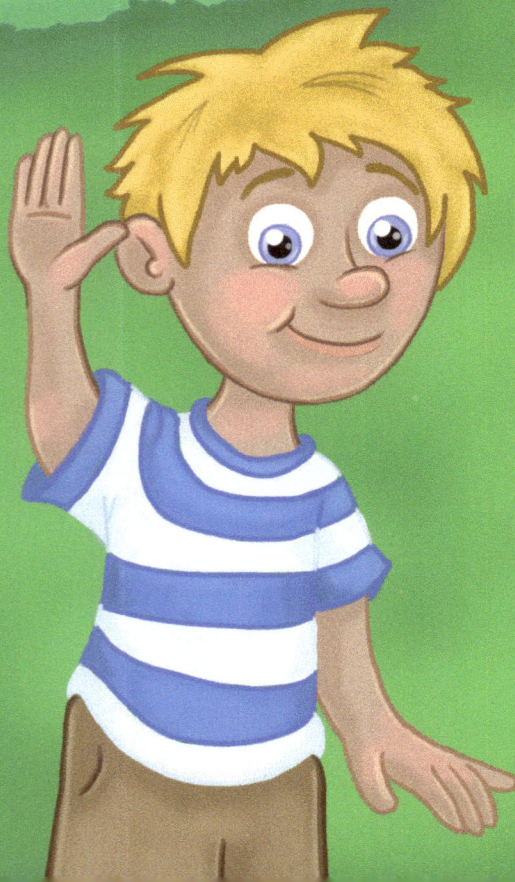

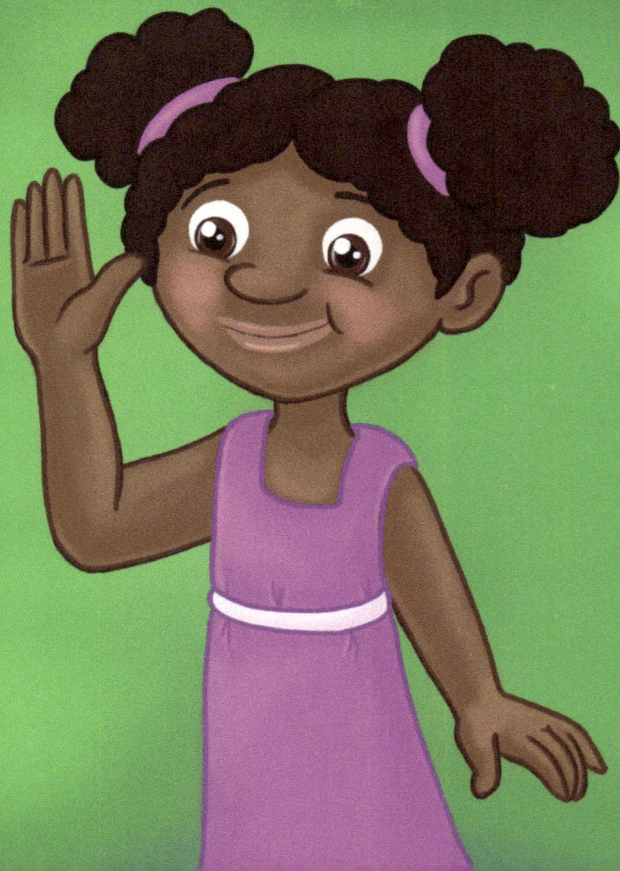

Children live all over the world. All children have a body that is unique and special. Each child has the right to keep their body safe.

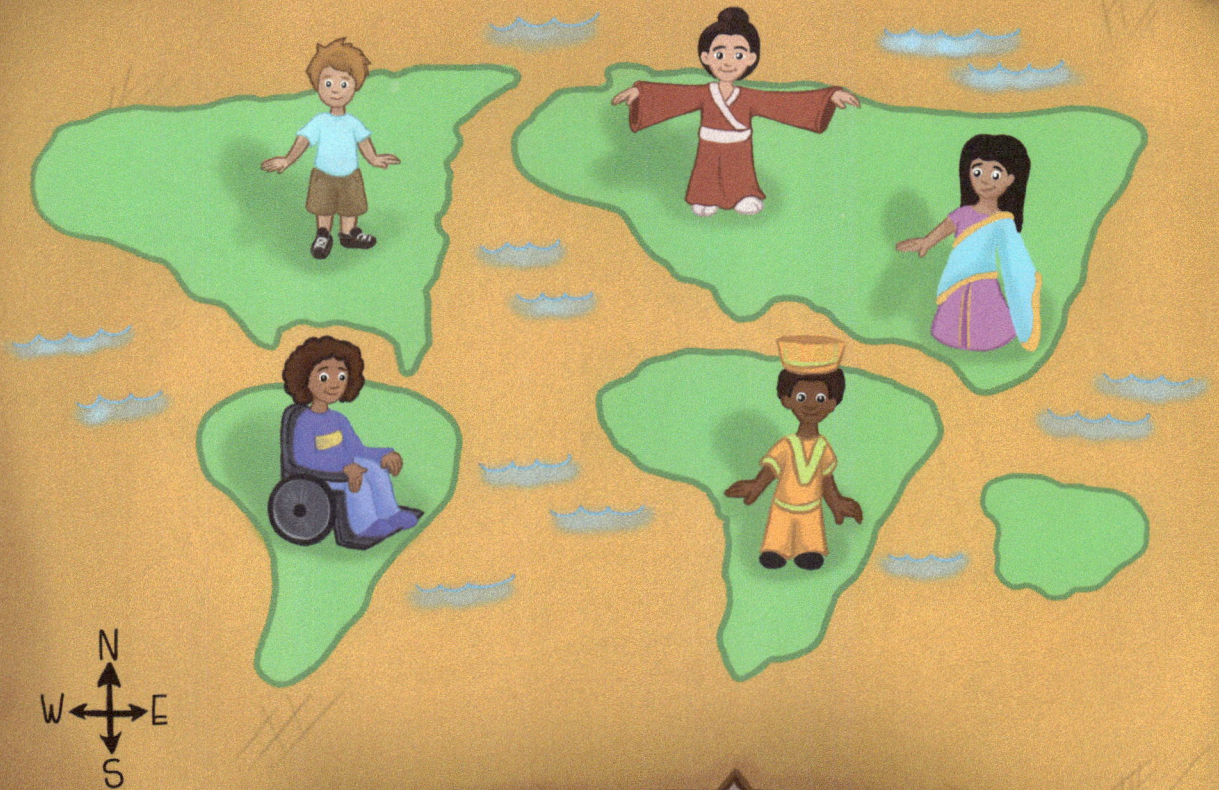

Boys

Girls

eye

ear

mouth

nose

neck

arm

chest

breasts

stomach

stomach

hand

butt

butt

thigh

testicals

leg

vagina

penis

foot

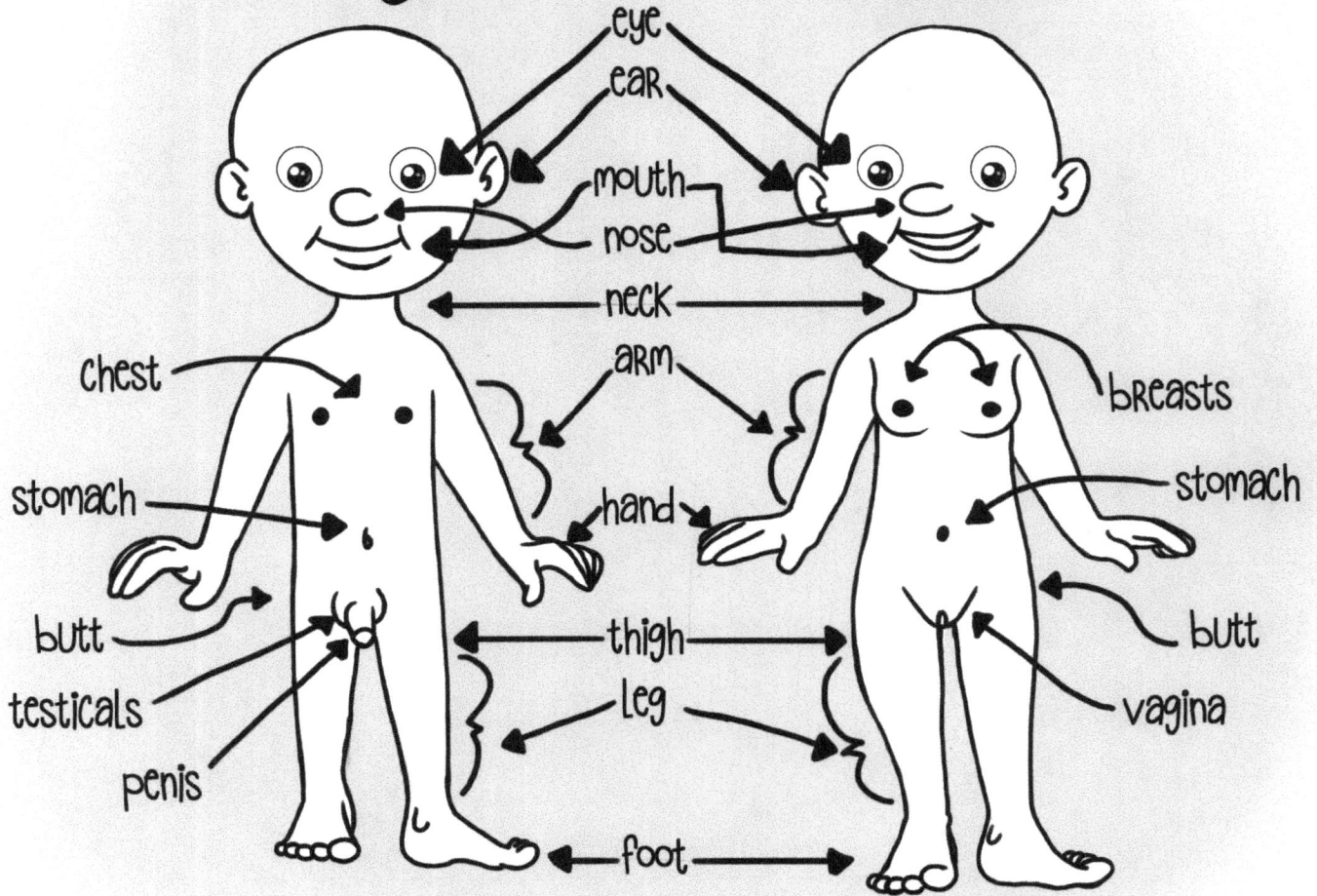

Your body is made up of parts. Some of your body parts are private. Private means that those body parts belong to only you. Let's learn about your body parts.

6

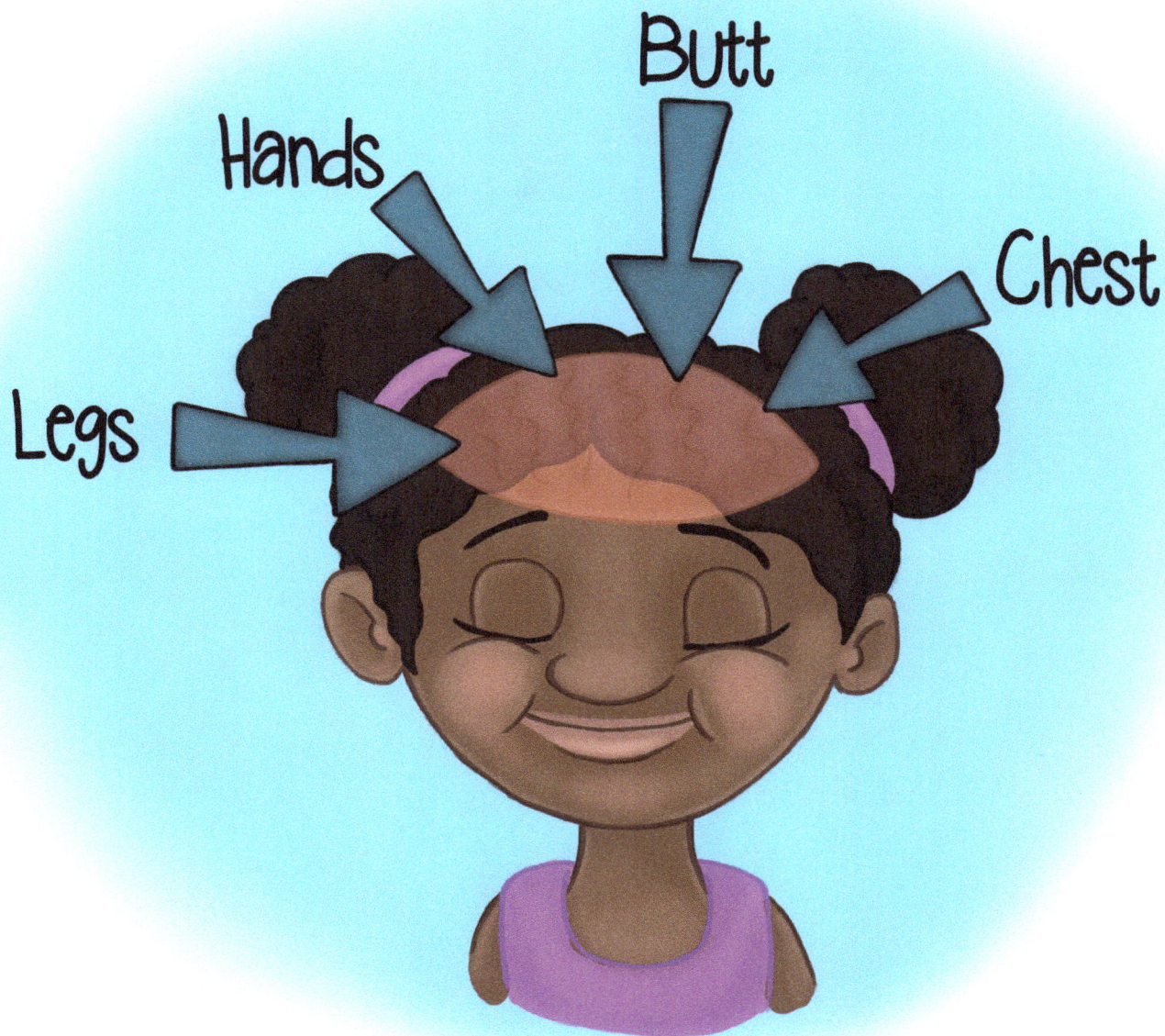

It is important to remember all the names of your body parts. Do not feel embarrassed to call your body parts by their real names because everyone has them.

Everyone has personal space for their body. Your personal space is the area around your body just like you were wearing an invisible hula-hoop. Respecting others' personal space by not getting too close to them is very important.

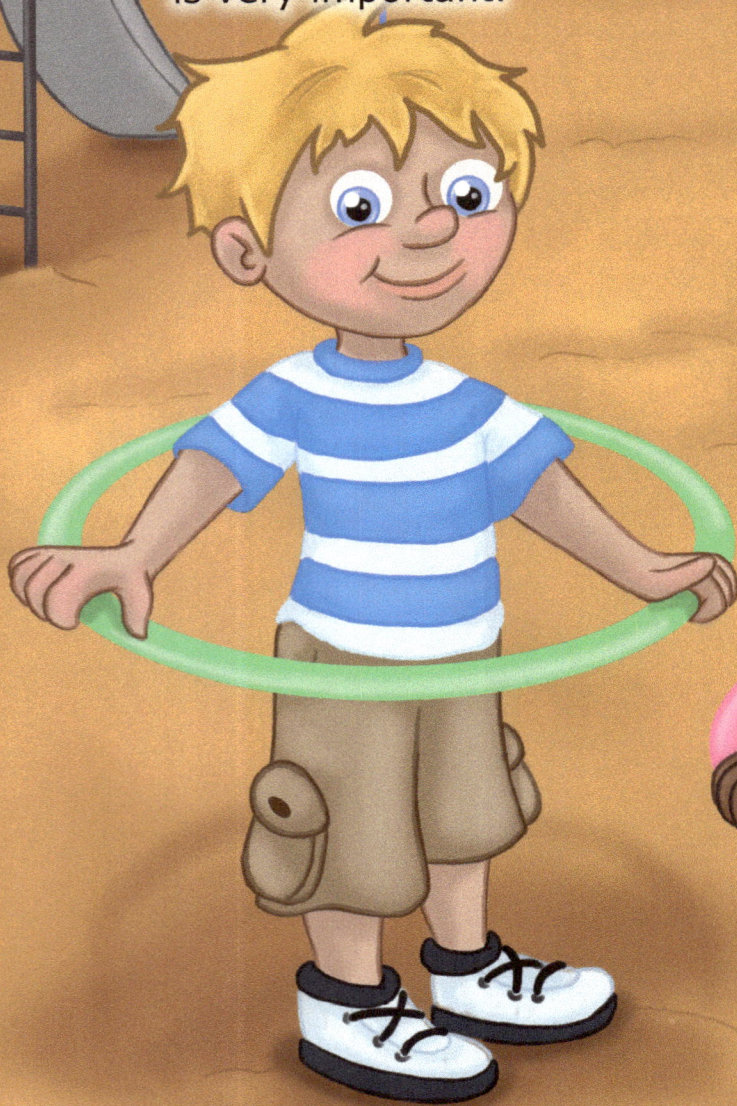

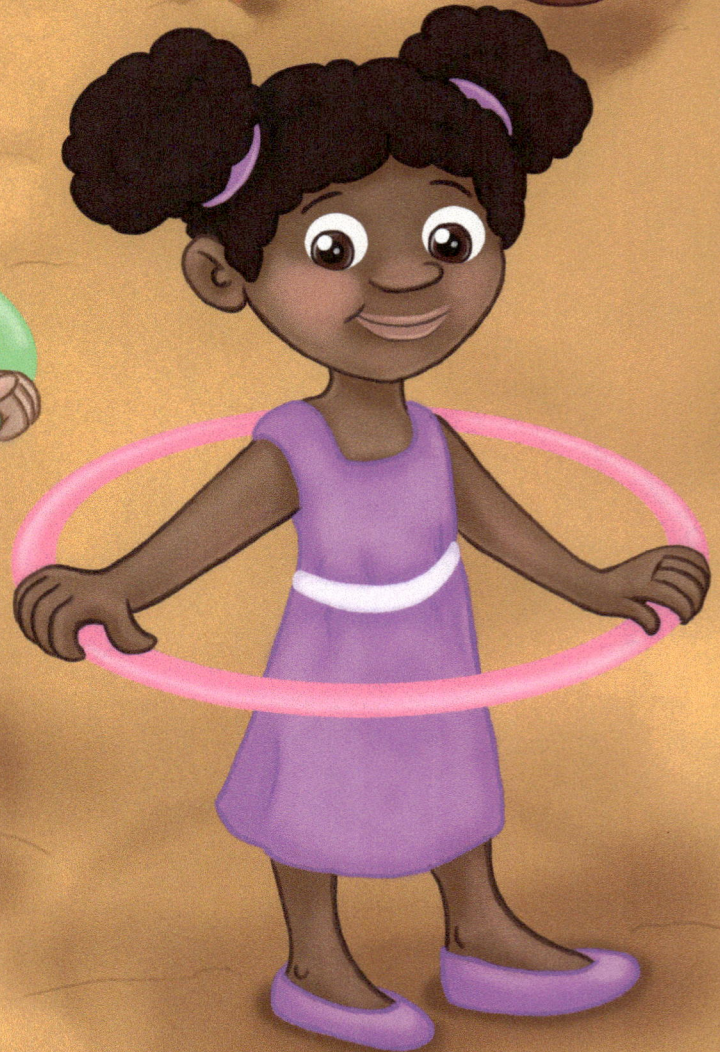

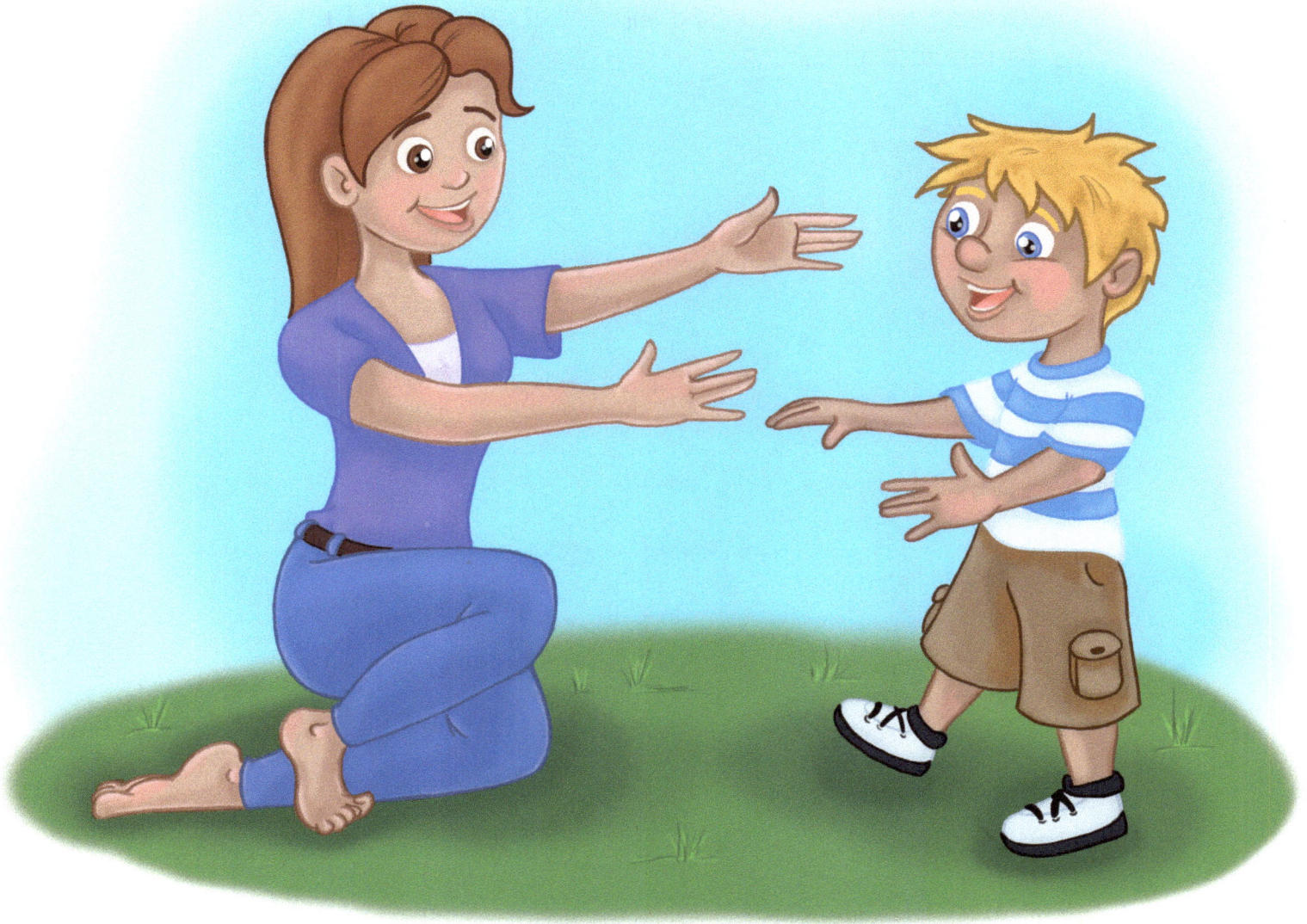

It is important not to go in anyone else's personal space without asking them first.

Some of your body parts are Stop Zones and some of your body parts are Go Zones.

Go Zones are your body parts that are okay for others to touch and see.

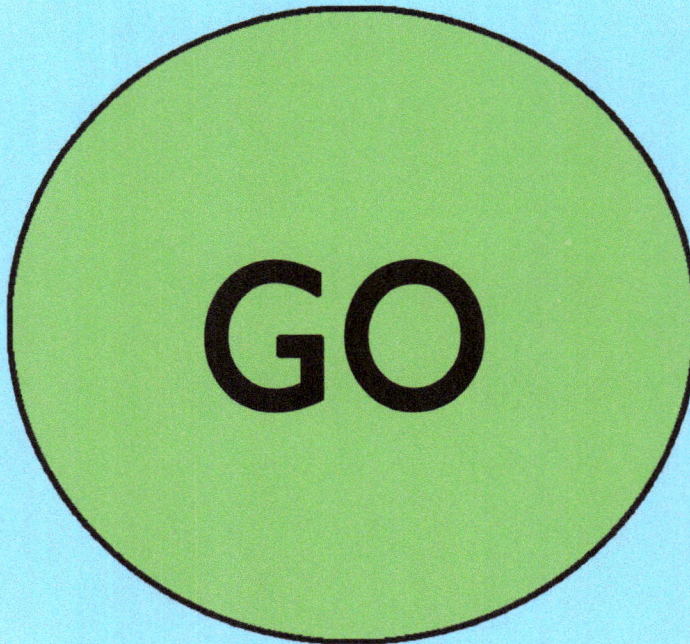

GO

Stop Zones are your private body parts that no one should touch or see except you. They are the body parts that are covered by a bathing suit when you go swimming. Even if someone asks you to see or touch your Stop Zones it is not okay because they are private.

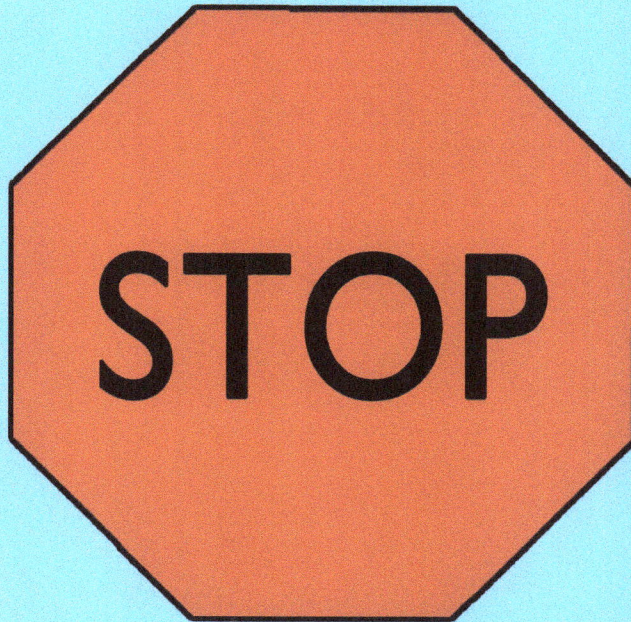

STOP

Boys

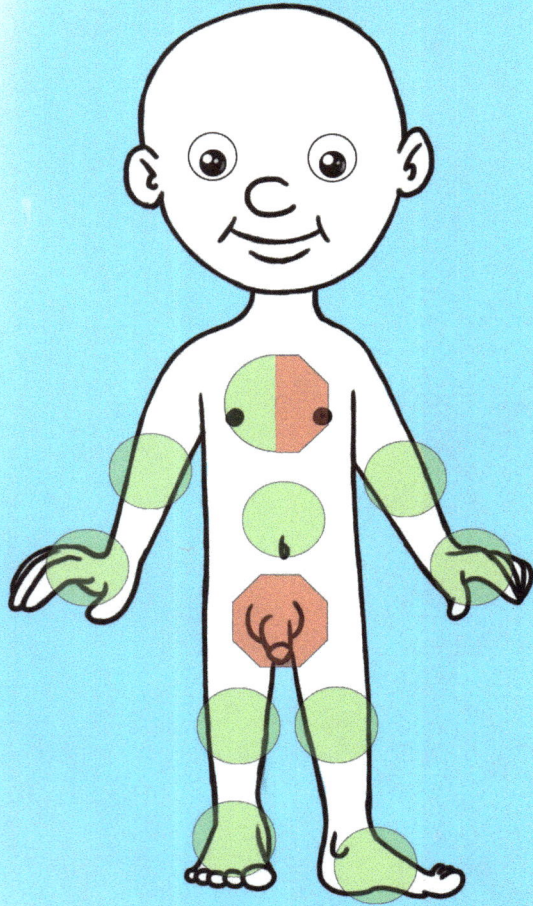

Girls

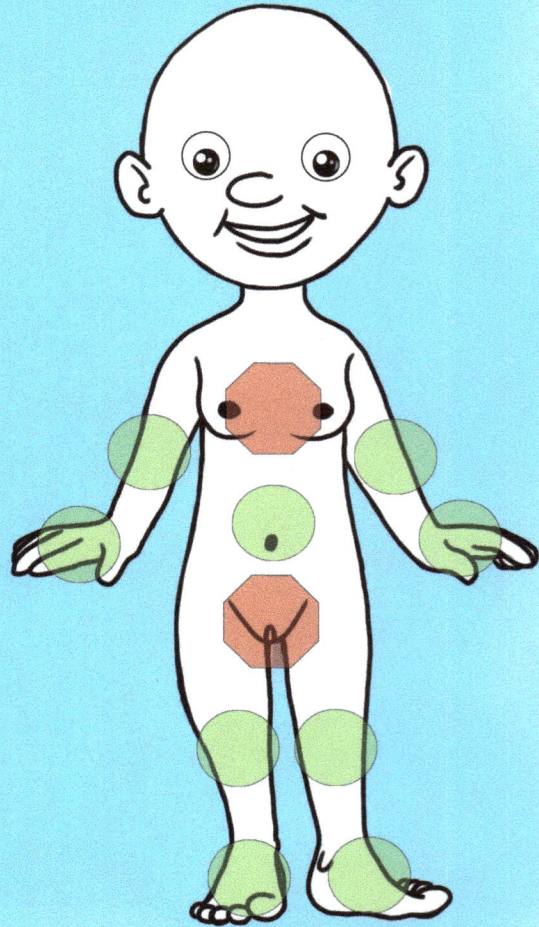

These are your Stop and Go Zones.

Stop Zones = **Red**
  Private body parts that are not safe for others to see or touch.

Go Zones = **Green**
  Body parts that are safe for others to see or touch.

  A boy's chest is both a Stop and a Go zone because it is safe for a boy to show his chest when he goes swimming, but it is not safe for others' to touch his chest because it is a private body part.

Everyone has an invisible "UT-OH" meter inside their body. Your "UT-OH" meter goes off when you feel unsafe. When your "UT-OH" meter rises your heart may beat fast, your stomach may hurt, or you may feel sweaty. It is important to listen to your invisible "UT-OH" meter so that you can keep yourself safe.

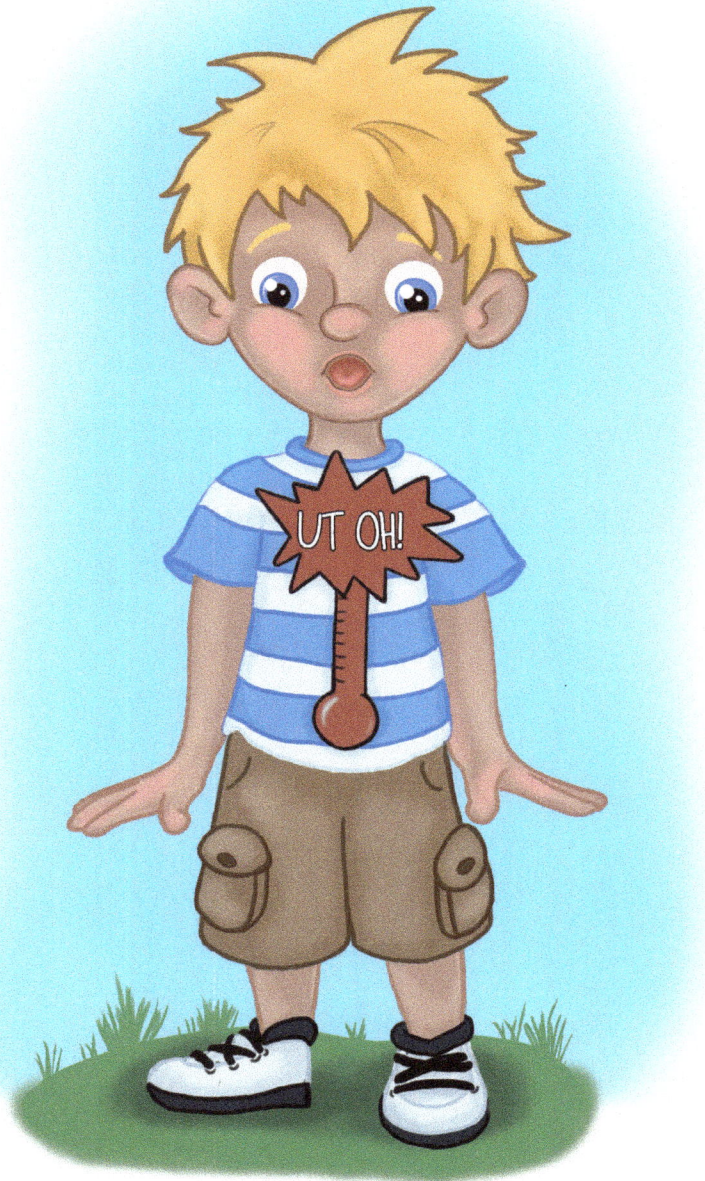

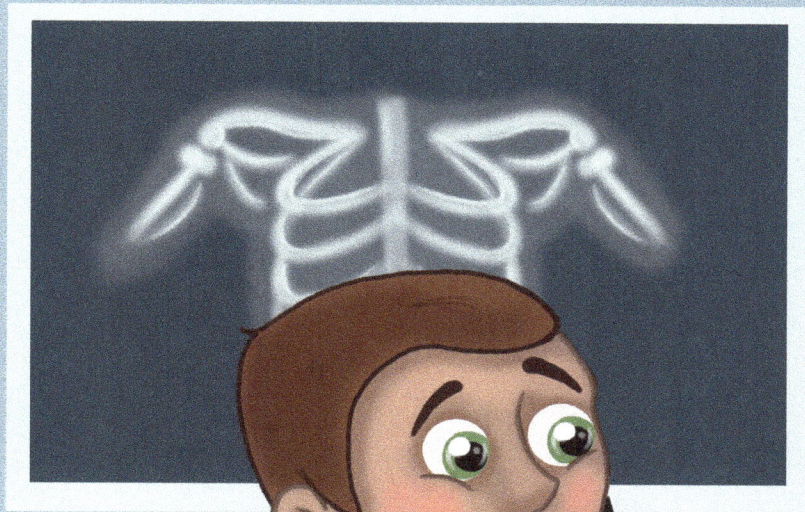

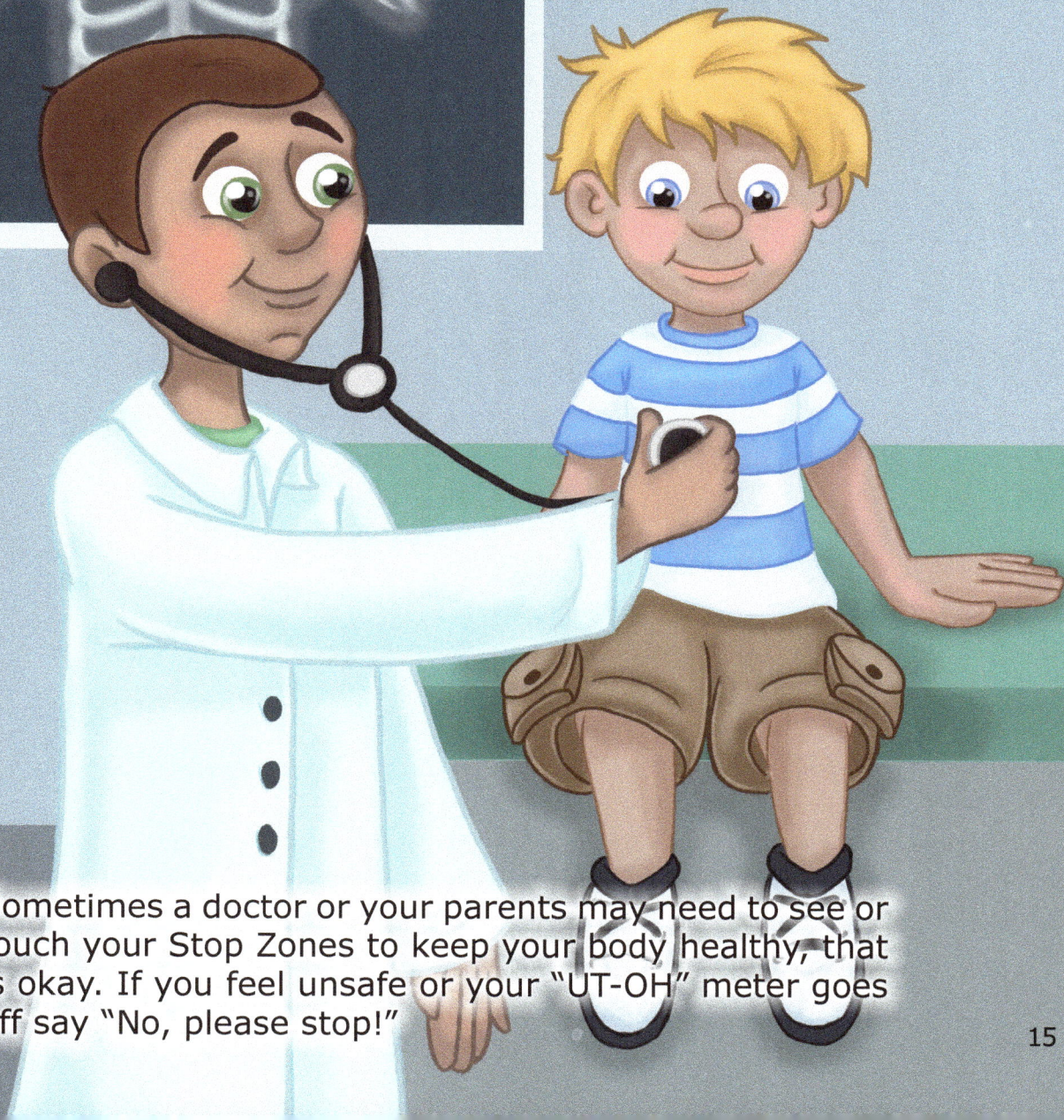

Sometimes a doctor or your parents may need to see or touch your Stop Zones to keep your body healthy, that is okay. If you feel unsafe or your "UT-OH" meter goes off say "No, please stop!"

Sometimes people may try to trick you into being unsafe with your body. These tricks may make your "UT-OH" meter go off. Tricks and touches on your Stop Zones may come from strangers or people you trust like your family or friends. No matter who touches your Stop Zones it is always okay to say "No, please stop!" You are smart and need to watch out for tricks to keep your body safe!

These are some of the tricks that someone may do when they want to see or touch your Stop Zones:

~ Give you a gift or food as a trade
~ Tell you that the touches are okay to do
~ Pretend it was an accident
~ Make you feel like the touches are your fault
~ Show you their private body parts
~ Ask you to touch their private body parts
~ Touch you when you are alone or sleeping
~ Tell you to keep the touches a secret
~ Try to scare or threaten you not to tell
~ Try to peek at your body when you are changing or showering
~ Pretend the touches are a game
~ Pretend that you are their special friend

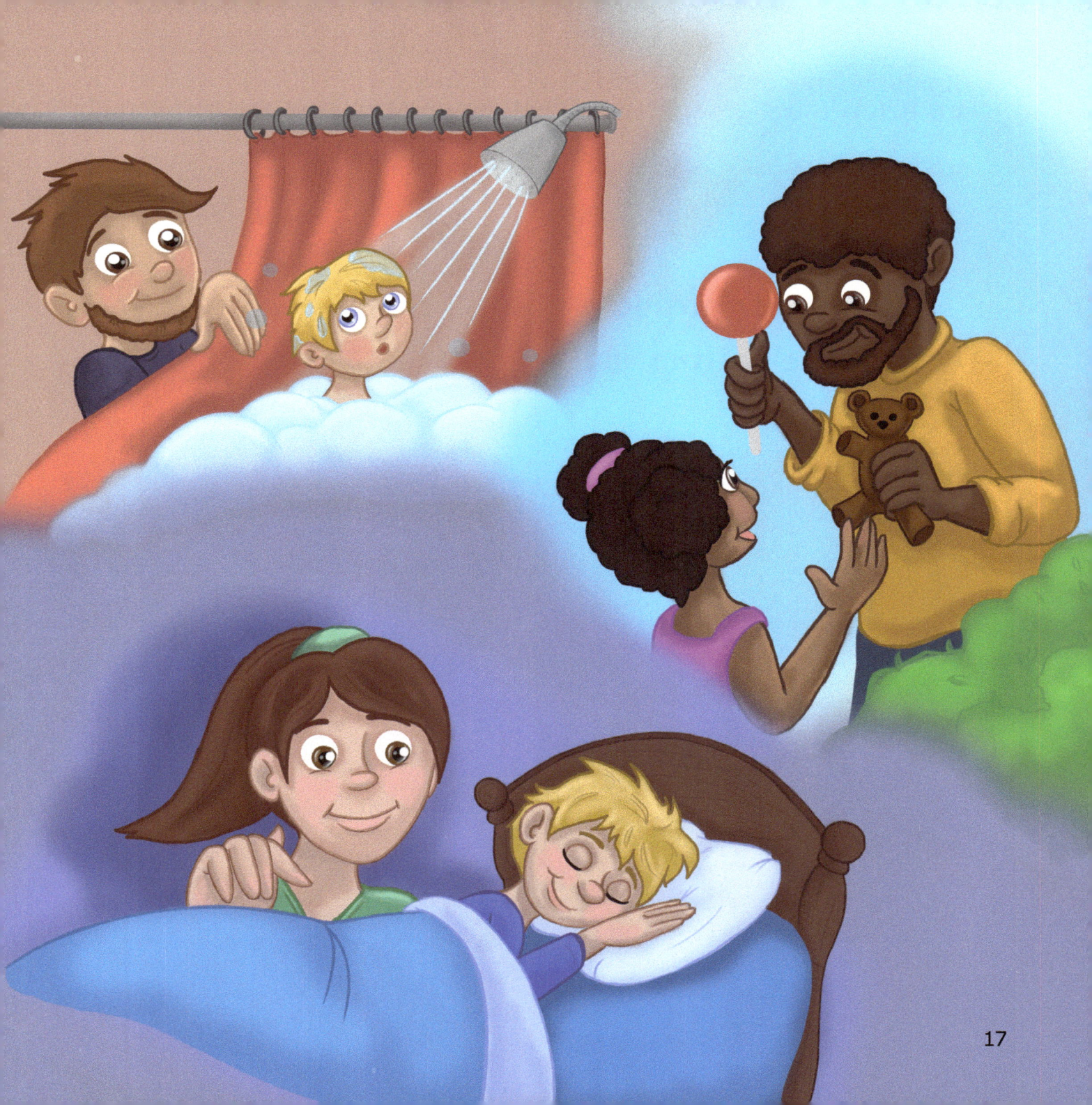

If anyone touches your Stop Zones or makes your "UT-OH" meter go off follow these safety steps. First, say "No, please stop!" Second, run away. Third, tell an adult you trust. You can tell your parents or grandparents.

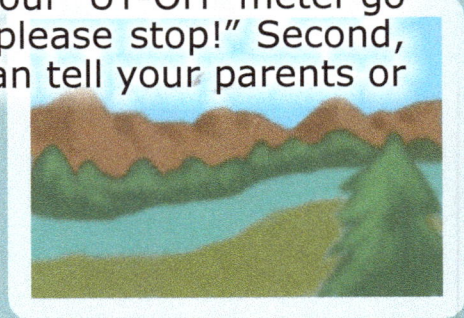

We are very proud of you for telling us.

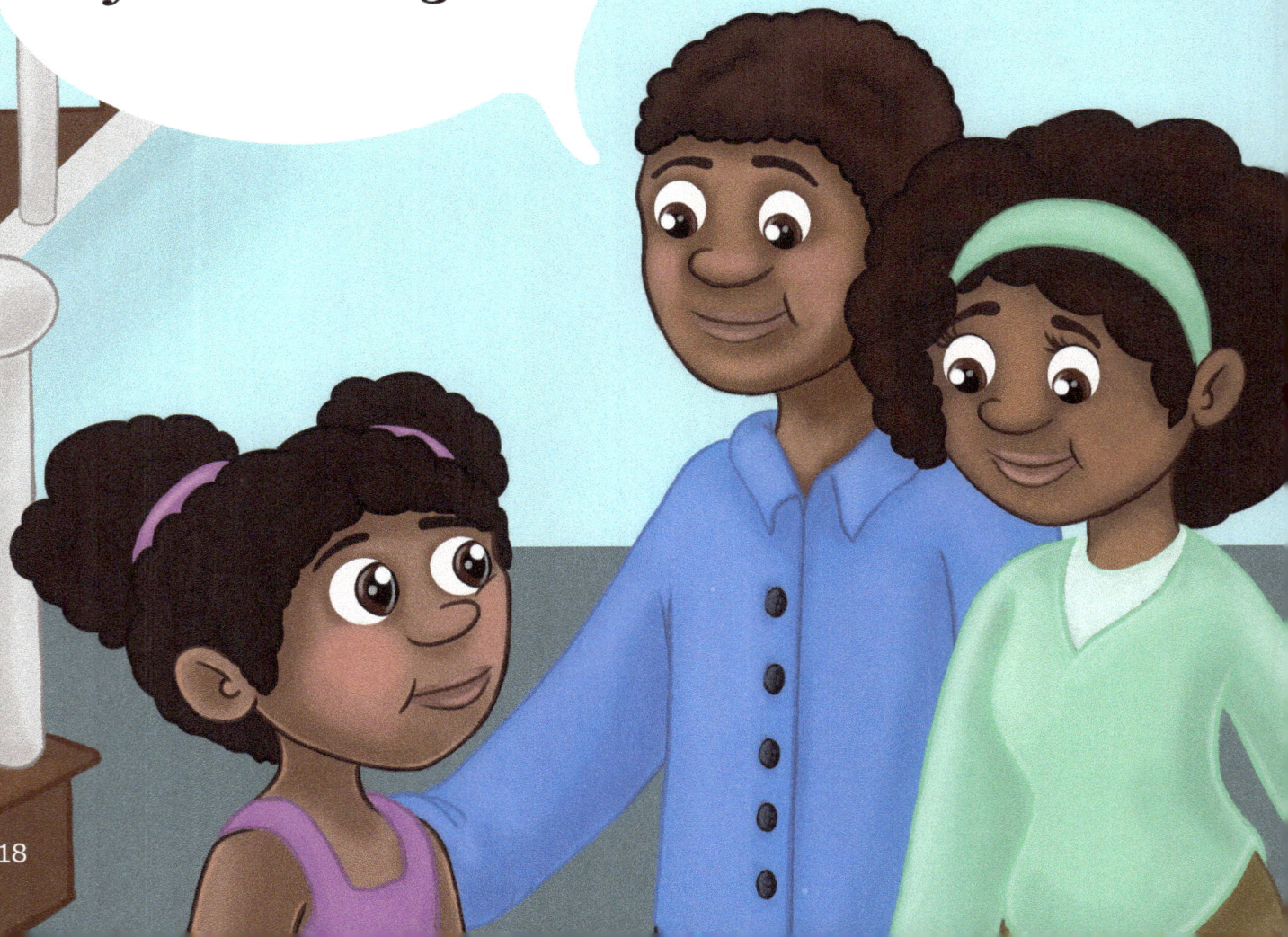

You can also get help by telling your teacher, coach, pastor, or the police.

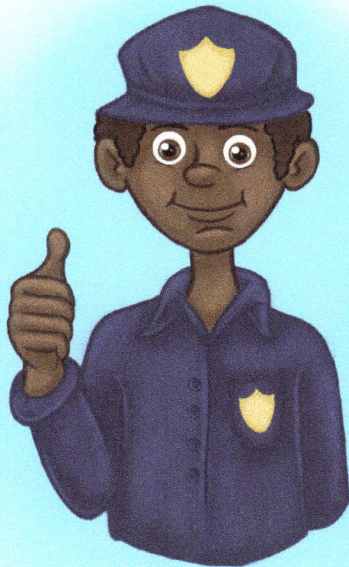 Police

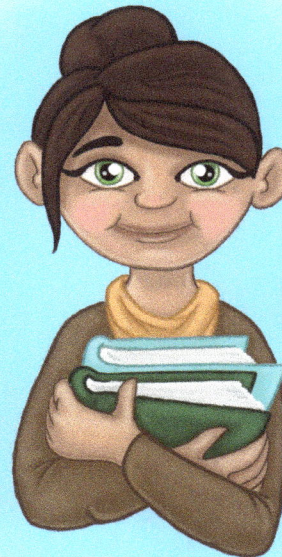 Teacher

Coach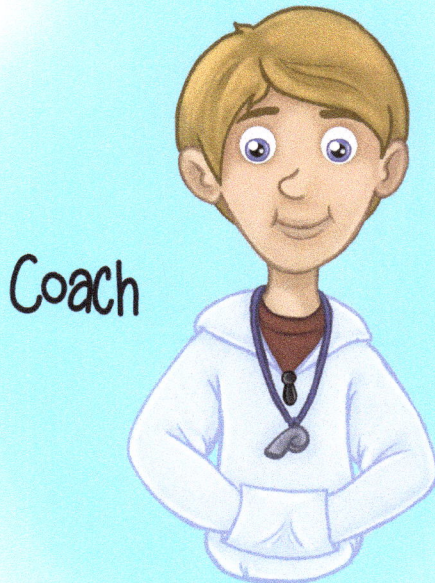

Pastor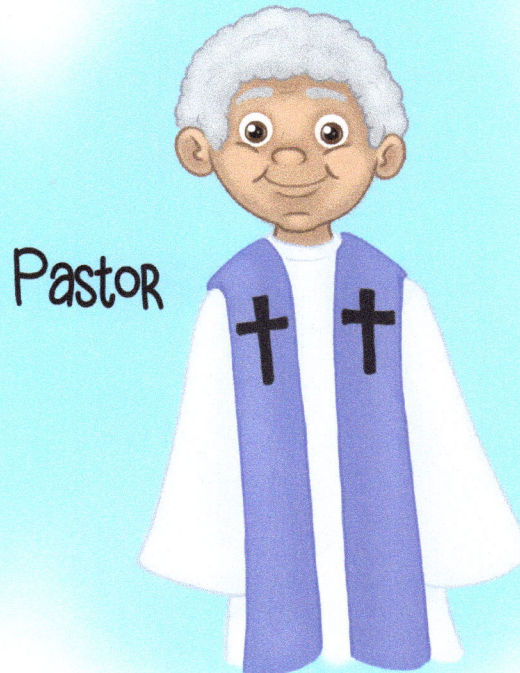

19

When you are telling a trusted adult, you can say "Someone touched my private body parts" or "Someone made me touch their private body parts." Remember to use the real name of your body parts. If the adult you tell doesn't believe you and help keep you safe, don't stop telling or give up! Tell another adult you trust until someone believes you and helps keep you safe!

Remember your body is special. So, let's keep our bodies safe!

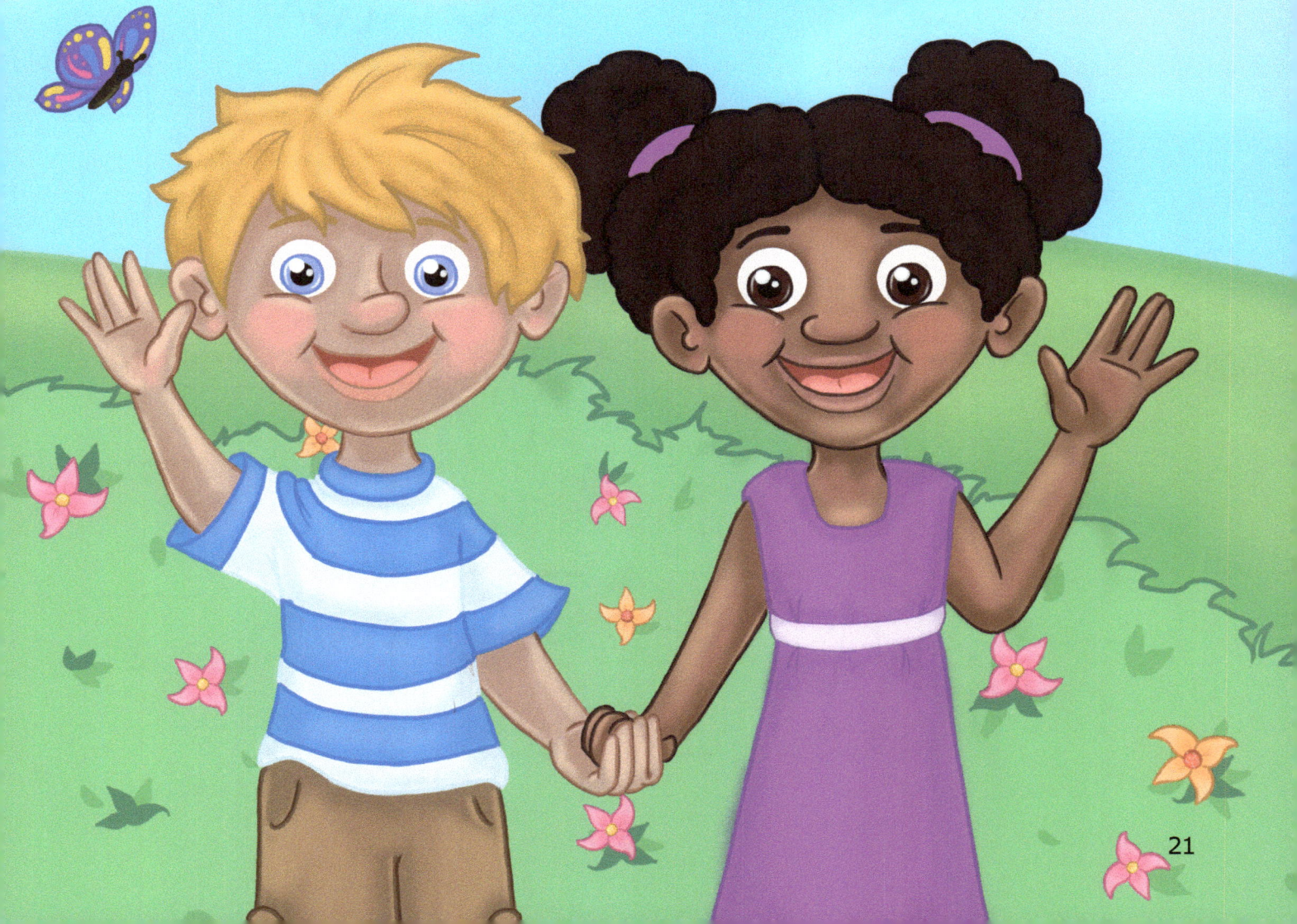

Zack and Zoie Safe Zones™
Safety Quiz

1.) Please label the body part names

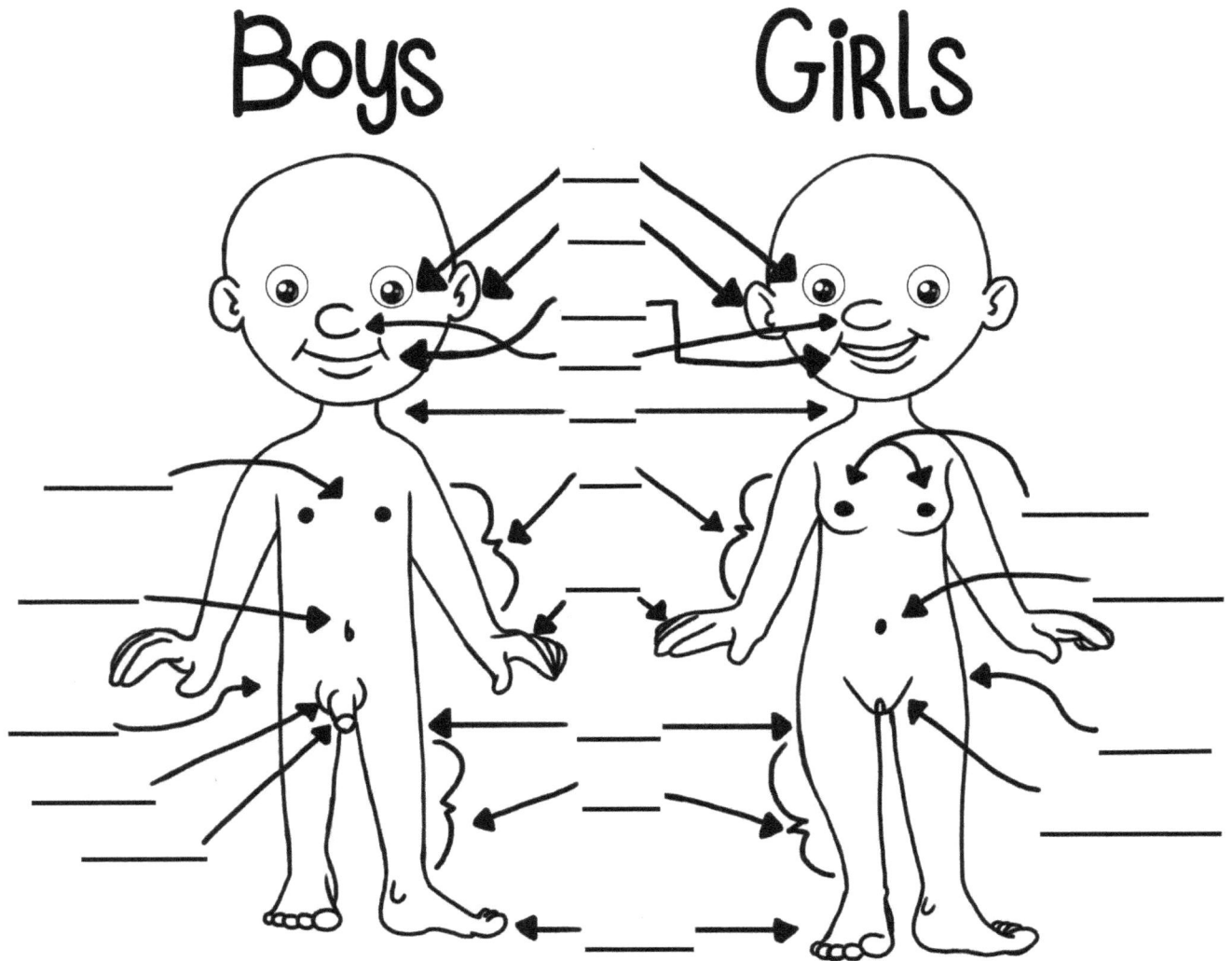

Boys

Girls

Zack and Zoie Safe Zones™
Safety Quiz

2.) I can say "No" to touches that make my "UT-OH" meter go off.

    a.) True   b.) False

3.) Circle the "tricks" someone may use to touch or see your Stop Zones.

    a.) give me a toy or present   c.) threaten to hurt me or someone else

    b.) pretend the touches are a game   d.) all of the above

4.) Fill in the blank for the Safety Steps.

    1.) Say "_____!"

    2.) _____ away.

    3.) Tell _____.

www.ingramcontent.com/pod-product-compliance
Lightning Source LLC
Chambersburg PA
CBHW041431270326
41934CB00022B/3500